Don't Blow Up Just Yet

A guide to Confronting the Menance of Anxiety in Girls and Women using Ancient Natural Therapies

Portia Cruise

© 2019 Portia Cruise

All rights reserved.

You are welcome to join the Fan's Corner, here

Disclaimer
The advice and strategies found within may not be suitable for every situation. This work is sold with the understanding that neither the author nor the publisher is held responsible for the results accrued from the advice in this book.

Dedication

This work is dedicated to Poje and Ses, without whose help, this book would not have come to light.

Table of Content

Getting Help, Where to Go

Alternative Treatments for Anxiety

1. *Aromatherapy*

2. *Cannabidiol Oil (CBD oil)*

3. *Herbal Teas*

4. *Herbal Supplements*

5. *Spending Time with Pets*

Natural Products for Anxiety Treatment

Other Effective Non-Herbal Techniques

Anxiety is Not Just About Doom

Anxiety is a global phenomenon and one of the symptoms associated with depression. Everyone experiences anxiety in varying degrees as a result of the activities we do which can have an effect on our physical and mental health. Our state of anxiety can be positive or negative, when anxiety is positive, it helps us manage situations that may have been devastating, like preparing for an interview, giving a public speech and involved in an emergency. The body uses anxiety in such situations to heighten our response rate and gives us that extra adrenaline to prepare better and deal with the situation appropriately. Without anxiety, the body would have difficulty handling the situation.

Anxiety can exhibit physical symptoms like increased heartbeat, sweaty palms, muscle tension, and headaches. This situation is usually short-lived and passes after the trigger or the cause has been removed. Anxiety can also have mental effects like insomnia, restless nights, exhaustion, chronic worry, lack of focus, and irritation. So for example, if you have lost a loved one, or have not heard from your child for a while, then it is natural that you will feel all these symptoms until the situation returns to normal or you may get closure if the worst possible scenario happened.

Anxiety becomes a case of mental health when it starts even when there is no trigger and it stays for a long time as soon as it has been triggered. It is believed that more than 40 million Americans suffer from anxiety and its related diseases. This book is, however, targeted at women and girls who suffer from stress and anxiety and are looking for natural remedies for treating it.

When a woman suffers from a continuous state of fear, nervousness, restlessness, and stress, she may be suffering from anxiety. Depression and stress tend to affect the body the same way anxiety does, but it does it in a far different degrees and effect. They all tend to occur as a result of the imbalance in the chemicals in the brain and neurotransmitters. Although often not considered a serious health issue by a lot of people, anxiety can affect the way we react to issues and even affect our interpersonal relationship with others. While there is no confirmed study as to how and why anxiety starts, it is believed that genetics plays a role and other contributing factors like change or loss of job, divorce, bills, risk of losing one's home or property, the loss of a dear relative or spouse, pressure at work, moving to a new apartment, changing school, preparing to get married, physical illness and environmental factors like living in an insecure area, can also sometimes lead to anxiety. Perhaps it could also be as a result of some changes in the body, pregnancy or even a miscarriage. Scientists also believe that some of these factors lead to loss of essential brain chemicals like serotonin, norepinephrine and dopamine neurotransmitters.

Improper drug use when taking certain medications for ailments like heart diseases, Alzheimer and diabetes are also believed to be among the major reasons why people have anxiety. Abuse of medication like sleeping pills can also have its effect. Women are more susceptible to having anxiety disorder than men in a lot of cases, mostly due to the hormonal changes that take place in their body. They also find it more difficult to deal with traumatic events and unpleasant situations in life.

Anxiety In Girls-Are You Affected?

Anxiety disorder in a woman becomes a problem when the woman panics or is anxious over trivial events or details. Men and Women tend to deal with anxiety differently, while men are able to shrug it off, women and girls tend to internalize it. Anxiety disorder and its symptoms are the number one health issue of women and girls in the USA and are the most common form of depression or other mental illnesses suffered by many American citizens.

Many women and girls who suffer from anxiety are unable to sleep properly, develop an overactive mind, and constantly worry over events that may not occur or can't change. When they are finally able to sleep, they achieve that in short duration with frequent intermittent breaks, leading to a distortion in their body balance. This can put a lot of stress and strain on the body. Scientists are sometimes not sure if it is insomnia that leads to anxiety or anxiety that leads to insomnia, whatever the case, both are detrimental to the health of the individual who suffers from it.

When the anxiety in a woman is allowed to fester and left untreated, it can escalate to chronic anxiety which can lead to severe consequences of an impaired immune system, frequent fatigue, nausea, heart palpitations, panic, and headaches. Periodic anxiety in the life of a woman is perfectly normal, it only becomes a matter of concern when it becomes too frequent especially in minor cases which often trigger an overreaction. It is advisable to seek medical help so that it does not become a full-blown mental disorder.

Although it is easy to suspect that a woman might be suffering from anxiety disorder based on the symptoms explained above, it is only a proper diagnosis from a medical practitioner that can confirm if a woman truly suffers from anxiety disorder or other ailments with similar symptoms like stress, depression, and mental breakdown.

Categories of Anxiety Disorder

Generalized Anxiety Disorder
People who suffer from this type of anxiety disorder have an exaggerated sense of worry over everything, including trivial issues even if there is nothing that provokes it.

Obsessive-Compulsive Disorder (OCD)

Obsessive- Compulsive Disorder (OCD) is an anxiety disorder that is usually associated with recurring, intrusive and unwanted thoughts often classified as obsessive. These thoughts tend to be repeated which is why it is called compulsive. People with this disorder worry and imagine the worse about anything and may often acknowledge their thoughts as silly all in a bid to get temporal relief. They may indulge in repetitive behaviors that include checking already locked doors, washing hands consistently, and washing their clothes every time because they worry about germs.

Panic Disorder

This type of disorder is characterized by unpredictable, intense fear and an overwhelming feeling of anxiety. This is majorly followed by repeated episodes of shortness of breath, heart palpitations, dizziness, and chest pain. When a person suffers from recurrent panic attacks or consistent fears for a period that exceeds more than a month, they are said to suffer from panic disorder.

Post-Traumatic Stress Disorder (PTSD)

A Post-Traumatic Stress Disorder (PTSD) is a type of anxiety disorder that can develop after the person has been exposed to a terrifying event or ordeal in which grave physical harm occurred or was threatened. Some traumatic events that can trigger PTSD include violent personal assaults, natural or human-caused disasters, accidents, or military combat.

Social Phobia (or Social Anxiety Disorder)
Humans as social animals tend to be conscious of how others perceive them. But people with social phobia or Social Anxiety Disorder are people who have an intense fear of being criticized, humiliated or scrutinized. It can be as mild as when the person has an insane fear of speaking in a formal or informal situation, eating or drinking in the company of people. This disorder is not discriminatory and does not care about the person's age, color, race, or level of education.

Specific Phobia Disorder
The social phobia is similar to the specific phobia and in this type of disorder, the person is unable to overcome the fear of doing a particular thing even though there is no need to fear and no matter the reassurances. Such fears may include phobia of heights, depths, water, taking flight and even being in a dark environment.

Leading Causes of Anxiety In Girls

There have been recognized leading causes of anxiety in women and girls, which have been noted over the years which are suspected to be the major causes of anxiety disorders. As the number of people affected by its effects continues to increase, scientists are beginning to take a more critical look at various methods of controlling and managing this problem, using modern day medical science. Although, the findings are so far not yet quite as definite as is common with a lot of mental illness and certain factors are known to increase the risk of suffering from anxiety disorder.

A person is unlikely to develop anxiety disorder from just one cause. It is generally believed that many people develop anxiety disorder from a combination of complex factors that form part of the causes and risk factors. As with other forms of mental illnesses, scientists are not able to confidently say what causes anxiety, but the following situations are found to be the major suspects.

Inherited

Anxiety and its effects tend to differ from one family root to another. This means that certain families are more likely to have anxiety disorder than others, which suggest that anxiety can be transferred from a parent to a child. People with first-degree relatives or family members with anxiety disorders, like a parent, have a higher risk of showing symptoms of anxiety disorders themselves.

Brain Chemicals

To function properly and respond adequately to issues, certain chemicals have to be released in the brain to the different sections that need it, and these chemicals have to be released in the right proportion based on how the brain interprets signals sent to it. So for every situation, the brain gets a measure of these different chemicals and a different measure and composition when the situation changes. When a condition that requires a person to be anxious occurs, the brain receives these various chemicals that help the person respond to that situation. The problem occurs, however, when a person with anxiety disorder begins to get a dose of these chemicals more frequently than is normal, especially when there is no known trigger to justify the release of these chemicals at the time they occur. These chemicals, which play a role in the development of anxiety disorders, are called neurotransmitters and they are the chemical messengers of the brain. When there is a low level of these neurotransmitters such as serotonin, dopamine, and norepinephrine, they cause a wrong signal of perceived danger to be transmitted to the brain.

Environment

The environment can also play a role in triggering the anxiety level in certain individuals, especially if those individuals experience stressors or triggers that was traumatic for them. The environment could be detrimental to a positive or negative flow of anxiety. A healthy environment could play a soothing role in decreasing the chances of triggering anxiety disorder or unnecessary worries.

Anxiety Triggers And Risk Factors

Women are far busier today than they have ever been. They juggle with work and career, relationships, volunteering at church, managing the home, and lots of other activities which puts them under a lot of pressure. These pressures also increase the chances of stress and make them susceptible to anxiety. Women and girls also tend to secretly compete among themselves and compare their lives with their peers and when they feel they are falling short, they put undue pressure on themselves eventually increasing the risk of anxiety.

Several factors combine to trigger a woman into a state of anxiety, as we have earlier identified three of the leading causes of depression and anxiety.

Sometimes, the daily routines of life cause us to be anxious. Even simple situations like what college to go to, where to hold our next birthday party, are we ready to get married, how do I meet the deadline on a project and numerous day to day activities can have its contributory effect. And with women and girls engrossed in a lot of activities nowadays, coupled with less time, they often don't have enough rest and care for themselves. They also do not do sufficient exercises, especially if every day of their week was hectic.

Women are also frequently burdened with the activities of the home, which is usually combined with the extra pressure to prove that they can perform at the same level as their male counterpart, this can also contribute to the person developing anxiety.

Another culprit when it comes to anxiety in women and girls has to be hormonal fluctuations, which tends to coincide with the period of the month when a woman is seeing her menstrual cycle. This is considered a biggie because this tends to occur in women and girls at least once in a month. This may also be associated with changes in her body structure, weight, wrinkles and other physical changes which can be perceived as not being desirable or going out of the present trend or fashion. So a normal gain in weight, which can be as a result of age, childbearing or poor diets can trigger a state of anxiety in a woman. Although hormonal fluctuations are not voluntary, the reaction of many women and girls to such hormonal fluctuations is what leads to anxiety tends to be self-inflicted.

Certain illnesses, as well as the drugs used in treating them, can sometimes lead to mood disorders as well as anxiety. Ailments like heart diseases, thyroid disorder, high blood pressure, stroke, high cholesterol, and cancer can make some women and girls anxious about their life. Although not considered as drugs, alcohol and caffeine are also considered common causes of anxiety and nervousness. Some prescription drugs, over-the-counter sleeping pills, anti-depressant and cigarette smoke containing nicotine can also affect the neurotransmitter function of the brain enough to trigger anxiety in some people. Certain irritations from toxins in the environment are suspected to also lead to a risk of anxiety disorder and irrational fear.

Poor diets and nutritional deficiencies are other causes of anxiety. Mood changes and disorder are also believed to be associated with nutritional deficiency and poor eating habits, which can lead to fatigue. A balanced diet is important for anyone who stands a risk of suffering from anxiety, that means eating less over-processed food and focusing on foods that increase the amount of fiber and other nutrients needed in the body.

One of the major reasons people become anxious is when they suddenly realize that they have a pile of work unattended to after haven procrastinated, thereby exposing them to a high level of stress when trying to meet up with deadlines. When a task that is supposed to be done with ease is put off or delayed to until a much later time unnecessarily, it adds to the pressure which can lead to an extra exertion when trying to meet up with the set date of delivery leading to a snowball of their anxiety over time.

Stress is a major cause of anxiety and is usually the first stage before the anxiety sets in. Stress is not always negative because it is what helps the body to amass the strength to deal with situations that seem tricky and difficult. When such stress is not properly managed and is sustained, it can also lead to a state of anxiety.

Symptoms
These are signs that are usually displayed by individuals who suffer from anxiety disorder which tends to vary depending on the genetic makeup of the person and severity of the symptoms. Most types of anxiety disorders have similar or general symptoms, before distinguishing the symptoms into any of the different types of anxiety disorders. These symptoms can be classified into behavioral, cognitive, physical and psychological symptoms.

Physical Symptoms
- Frequent Urination
- Aches and pains in the body
- Nausea
- Insomnia
- Lightheartedness and Fatigue
- Numbness or tingling feet and hands
- Difficulty in swallowing
- Sweating and headaches
- Increased shock response
- Fear and trembling
- Restlessness and dizziness

- Breathing difficulty, increased pulse rate, increase heart rate, heavy breathing

Behavioral Symptoms:
- Worry excessively about every aspect of life
- Worry even when there is very little trigger
- Excessive and exaggerated course of unrealistic worry almost throughout the day and week
- Exaggerated worrying for a circumstance that is unwarranted

Psychological Symptoms:
- Worry over anything, whether big or small
- Highly pessimistic about things improving
- Irritability
- Feelings of unworthiness
- Exaggerated perspective of problems
- Agitation
- Mood swings

Cognitive Symptoms:
- Mind going blank
- Short attention span
- Memory Loss
- Trouble concentrating
- Difficulty making decisions
- Muscle tension
- Unable to stay calm and still

Effects of Anxiety in Girls and Their Symptoms

Women and girls are 60% more likely to be diagnosed with anxiety and the triggers for men also tend to be different from that of women- at least some of it. Some effects of anxiety in girls include:

Depression

It is believed that more than 20% of women who suffer from anxiety also end up with depression which is one of the reasons why anxiety must be treated as soon as it is detected. Depression is a more serious ailment which can have very grave consequences. People who suffer from depression tend to view life as being unfair, harsh and cruel to them, which tends to increase their rate of suicide. Many people who are depressed find themselves alone and lost in their thoughts, worries, and fears. Anxiety, stress, and depression make those who suffer from it to be unable to focus and are easily weighed down by their stressors.

Sleeping Problems

Anxiety can lead to loss of sleep in girls who suffer from anxiety disorder. Sleeping helps the body and brain to rest from the daily stressful routine and the body is able to regulate the different hormones in the body and help the person stay refreshed. However, when the body is denied the sleep it deserves, the body reacts. A person who does not get enough sleep is likely to get touchy, fatigued, paranoia and restless. If this continues for a long time, it can increase the risk of having more severe ailments like stroke, high blood pressure, and stress.

Emotional Stress

Anxiety also increases the emotional distress in women and girls to very high levels. Such emotional distress leads to frequent anger, irritation, and hostility. The emotional distress also results in irrational fears of both known and unknown perceived consequences of events and outcomes. This leads to the person being sad, depressed and apprehensive over little things.

Changes in Physical Attributes

Anxiety can make the body react to real and perceived dangers by changing the normal working of the body which increases the heartbeat, causes muscle tension and indigestion.

Fatigue and Exhaustion

The emotions of an individual who suffers from anxiety can put a physical drain on the person and this can lead the individual to become tired as a result of the extra work that the body has to do. Many women and girls report that they tend to feel fatigued and are left exhausted after every episode. Fatigue also reduces the energy level in women and girls, which makes it difficult for them to be involved in self-help activities that could have helped to alleviate the feelings of anxiety. Important activities like exercising, camping, and other physical activities become difficult to do because of exhaustion caused by anxiety.

Other effects of anxiety include:

- Unable to handle responsibilities
- Frequent family and marital problems
- Low capacity to act quickly or accurately
- Inability to interact normally with others
- Agoraphobia (fear of being in public places)
- Low level of motivation
- Frequent Suicidal Thoughts and Behaviors
- Palpitations or Elevated Heart Rate
- GI Distress /IBS /Diarrhea
- Frequent Flashes
- Sudden Changes in Body Temperature

How You Can Help

People with anxiety require all the help that they can get, even if they do not admit or know it themselves. If you know anyone that requires some sort of help based on the signs you have observed pertaining to anxiety disorder, then you have to do whatever you can to help that person.

When a person has suffered any form of trauma in their lives and suddenly begin to seek solitude and isolation even though the person wasn't always like that, then anxiety which could lead to depression may be setting in. If this situation describes anyone you know, even it is just a neighbor around you, a friend, in the church, colleague, even someone you know from a distance, you can take a pause from what you are reading right now and please reach out to that person. Such persons may just be yearning for someone to genuinely show them some concerns and lend them a helping hand.

Anxiety disorder is likely to require therapeutic help, which may mean that one of the ways you can help is by convincing the person to go and seek medical help from experts. Because many people do not like to admit that they have anxiety disorder or any disorder for that matter, they delay going to seek medical help for as long as possible, sometimes leaving it until a lot of damage has been done. No matter the good intentions you may have towards persons suffering from anxiety disorder, you are not likely to be able to cure them on your own.

One of the roles you will need to play when helping a person with anxiety disorder will be to get them to the clinic as soon as possible, so that they can begin their medication at once. You can offer to assist with childcare when they are away on the visit or even offer to follow them there, especially on their first appointment so that they do not develop cold feet along the way. More likely than not, Cognitive-Behavioral Therapy (CBT) will be the starting point. This therapy has proven to be the most effective treatment for anxiety in a lot of cases. It mostly involves learning to solve problems, and avoiding some of the triggers that lead to anxiety.

Sometimes, the therapy recommended may not involve drugs, but other forms of activities that may include exercises, massage to reduce stress and guided visual imagery. You can help by ensuring that the person actually does these things. You are more likely to succeed if you do that by actually encouraging the person rather than trying to force them to do it. There will be situations when you will need to disregard any form of resistance, and be firm, knowing that you are acting in their best interest and when they eventually pull through, they will come to appreciate you as a true friend who stood by them in their moments of vulnerability. Who wouldn't crave to have such a friend who looks out for us even when we resist and are too weak to even help ourselves especially in our darkest moments.

One trigger for anxiety in women and girls is when they procrastinate, in doing so, they discover that the activities that they could have handled earlier are left unattended to, they become anxious when trying to get them done. To help them, you can help them to stay focused by showing them how to prioritize different task and draw up a list of work they intend to do daily with specific periods of the day they should do them. You can try to get them to make that important phone call they have been putting aside or picking up some groceries from the supermarket or having that crucial discussion with her boss. Whatever the task may be, the more an anxious person puts aside what they intend doing, the higher the chances of them experiencing intruding thoughts of things yet undone. Ironically, the periods when they focus on those activities enables them to be distracted from the different stressors that can trigger their anxiety disorder.

Talking about distraction, other ways you can help someone with anxiety is by creating activities that will benefit both of you in the management of stress. Some recommended and effective stress management strategies that you can easily create at little or no cost can be dancing, listening to music, hanging out with friends, exercising, and watching a motivational movie. Some other activities include taking a long walk through the park, visiting the beach and fun centers. These activities will help the body use more oxygen and enable the brain to operate faster. Such simple techniques will not only help the person with anxiety to deal with the symptoms of anxiety, it also helps the person who is providing the support mentally.

You also help a person with anxiety by scrutinizing their eating habits and suggesting a more balanced form of diets that works for them. To handle difficult situations better, it is always important the mind and body are healthy, so a good diet that consists of lean proteins, fiber, fruits, grains, and vegetables have been found not only to be nutritious but also very helpful.

Another excellent way you can help someone with anxiety disorder deal is to show them how to be optimistic in life. People who suffer from anxiety disorder are often embarrassed by the symptoms they exhibit and often fear that the symptoms may be so obvious to people around them, especially when they are being watched, perhaps in a performance or presentation, or in social gatherings. For example, rather than spend time preparing for their client meetings, they may find themselves worrying about what tone of voice they should use if the client will notice their shaking fingers, sweaty palms, and tensed voice. You can help them to try to stay calm and positive, rather than focus on the negative things that may happen, you can assure them that everyone feels that way in one way or the other, that they are very capable of handling it.

Managing and Treating Anxiety
Anxiety disorder can sometimes be serious; enough to distort a person's way of thinking to the extent that it can affect the person's work, school, and general well-being. To recover from it, appropriate treatment has to be initiated as soon as possible. Proper treatment for anxiety takes into cognizance the different aspects of anxiety disorder and recommends treatments based on these aspects. Common aspects usually handled by therapist include:

1. Psychological Treatment
2. Medical Treatments for Anxiety
3. Anxiety Management Strategies

Psychological Treatment

This form of treatment involves speaking with the patient in a way that tries to help shape the person's thinking pattern so the frequent episodes of anxiety can be better controlled and irrational worries reduced. Psychological treatments come in various types and the manner of delivery differs from one to the other. Some forms of this therapy involve having a one-on-one session with the patient, while some others may prefer a peer group approach that helps prepare the participants on what to expect. Sometimes, a combination of the two systems is used. The types of Psychological treatments include:

1. Cognitive Behavior Therapy (CBT)
2. Behavior Therapy
3. e-Therapies

Cognitive Behavior Therapy (CBT)

This form of treatment is believed to be one of the most effective of the different types of anxiety treatment. It also has a lot of documented evidence to back it up. At the core of cognitive behavior therapy is the fact the things a person believes to be true is what can trigger their thoughts, which can then trigger in them the feelings that determine their behavior. It is a structured psychological form of treatments that acknowledges that the person's way of thinking (cognitive) and acts (behavior) is what affects the way the person feels. In CBT treatment, the practitioner helps the patient identify the behavioral patterns and thoughts that have a tendency to make you become anxious or inhibits you from getting better when you experience anxiety. As soon as the problematic patterns are identified, then changes can be recommended that will attempt to replace those patterns with new ones that tend to reduce anxiety and improve your coping skills.

This step usually involves doing away with pessimistic thinking pattern that usually involves believing things are usually worse than they really are. With CBT therapy, you are shown how to be more realistic in your thinking and focus more on solving problems. The therapist is likely to help find ways to actively avoid situations or circumstances that make you feel anxious, so that you are better able to face your fears and approach every situation in a more rational way.

After undergoing CBT, the patient is likely to find that she is better equipped to differentiate irrational worries from those that are not productive and lead to unnecessary anxiety that should be discarded, the patient will also learn how not to focus too much on worries, but instead focus more on solving problems. The training generally involves practicing breathing techniques, muscle relaxation, and positivity.

Behavioral Therapy

The behavior therapy is often combined with the CBT, which is why it is called the CBT, with the "B" standing for behavior, when trying to treat anxiety disorder or other forms of mental disorder. However, unlike the CBT, behavior therapy doesn't try to get the patient to change his thinking, instead it is more concerned with encouraging the patient to be more involved in activities that give more reward, pleasures and gives them a sense of satisfaction in an attempt to reverse the temptation to procrastinate on task and avoid the worry associated with it that makes the whole situation worse. Behavior therapy helps the victim learn how to cope with a fearful situation rather than just trying to run away from them.

e-Therapies

This type of therapy is not really so different from the aforementioned therapies above. Instead, it is the mode of delivery that is different. With the advancement in technology, it is only natural that the medical field also takes advantage of the various technologies available. The use of e-therapy allows practitioners to conduct consultation online with their patients. Most e-therapies or computer-aided psychological therapy use the principles of CBT or Behavior therapy when administering treatment on the patient. Because these forms of treatment tend to be structured, it becomes easy to deliver online without the need to see the patient in person.

The communication channel is usually via emails, instant messaging, via calls or SMS. The advantage of this approach is that you do not need to drastically change your schedule to be on the road and is particularly beneficial to those people who live far away from the therapist.

Medical Treatment for Anxiety
Although mental health practitioners believe that the use of psychological therapies remains the best form of treatment for people with anxiety, the patient sometimes has to be subjected to medical aids when the condition of the patient becomes severe. These drugs are administered with great caution while the patient is made to undergo observation to ensure there are no adverse reactions or abuse.

1. Antidepressant medication
2. Benzodiazepines

Antidepressant Medication
Antidepressant medications are designed to make the person with the disorder feel better and make it easier to manage their anxiety better even when there are no obvious symptoms of depression. Unlike psychological forms of treatment, they do not attempt to influence your way of thinking or alter your behavior, instead, they try to correct in the imbalance of brain's chemical called serotonin, noradrenaline and dopamine, used in the

transmission of messages between the nerve cells or neurons in the brain.

The doctor will determine the duration of the treatment based on how severe the symptoms are and how quickly the patient responds to treatment. Some are able to stop after a short time, while others have to keep taking it as an ongoing process. Antidepressants are also very useful for people with suicidal thoughts and help in reducing the likelihood of patient injuring themselves.

Usually, before administering these drugs, the doctor will find out if the patient has any allergies and discuss the side effects with them. Most of these side effects are dependent on the patient's physical fitness, state of health and general well-being. Common and possible side effects that some patients have reported include headache, dizziness, agitation, weight gain, low libido, and nausea. Most of the symptoms are short-lived as the body tries to adjust to the new drug that is being introduced into the body. Fortunately, antidepressants have been found to be effective and safe and are not known to be addictive.

Benzodiazepines
This class of drugs is sometimes referred to as minor sleeping pills and tranquilizers which help the patient relax and reduce tension. Unlike the antidepressant medications, they are not recommended to be used as long-term drugs, instead, they are used for short periods

of time or intermittently as part of a broader form of treatment and rarely as the first line of treatment because of their side effects which can leave the patient feeling dull, uncoordinated and hooked.

Anxiety Management Strategies

They are a wide range of strategies you can use to manage your anxiety. What works for one person may not work for others, and it can take some time before one can find the strategies that work best for you in the management of anxiety.

Anxiety management strategies can be used in combination with other strategies provided by professionals. Getting informed about the physiology of anxiety management, with concerns as to respond with a fight or a flight, as a way of dealing with impending danger is a very important aspect of dealing with and managing anxiety. People with anxiety are triggered in a manner that interprets harmless situations as dangerous.

Learn Proper Breathing Technique

This technique is for people who are anxious to breathe faster and take shallow breaths. This causes oxygenation, which increases the oxygen levels in the system and reduces the level of carbon dioxide in the blood. Not many people realize that carbon dioxide helps to regulate the reaction of the body to panic and anxiety. By learning to breathe properly when anxious, you are able to manually control and regulate the amount of oxygen and carbon dioxide in the blood. There are a couple of techniques for breathing properly, but all are geared towards slowing down the rate of breathing.

Learning Muscle Relaxation

A person with anxiety disorder is likely to have difficulty relaxing, which is why it is important to learn how to release the tension in the muscle. A common technique is to slowly tense and then releasing the various muscle groups in the body by holding the tension for a period of three seconds before releasing quickly.

Meditation

Meditation is another effective way of managing anxiety. Anxiety can make a person imagine the worst case scenario in every situation even when there is no sufficient evidence to back up such a pessimistic perspective. By practicing meditation, the person who suffers from anxiety is able to have a realistic view of a situation and stay in the present moment. It also helps them focus only on thoughts that are useful. Meditation works by slowing down racing thoughts, making it easier for the patient to manage stress and anxiety. Various forms of meditation styles are available, which can be combined with yoga and mindfulness.

Get Involved in Physical Activities

It is essential to stay active by getting involved with activities. Individuals who suffer from anxiety disorders can take advantage of these activities which can help reduce moments of anxiety and improve general well being like visiting locations that showcase nature, being in the company of family and friends who are able to assist in engaging in productive banters that helps to reduce boredom. It is also important to indulge in frequent exercises that help to burn up the chemicals that aid stress.

Maintain a Healthy Lifestyle

By eating a healthy diet, the body is able to get the minerals it needs to be able to help the muscles relax. Minerals like magnesium are particularly very important in getting the muscle tissues to relax. A magnesium deficiency tends to contribute to insomnia, depression, anxiety and improper regulation of the body system. The body also needs a sufficient dose of vitamin B and Calcium to ensure symptoms of anxiety are not exacerbated. Individuals with anxiety disorder should avoid stimulants like Nicotine and Caffeine that have the capacity to trigger adrenal glands that send out adrenaline, which is the predominant stress chemical. Where possible, your diets should consist of whole grain cereals, vegetables and dairy products that have low fats while avoiding foods with artificial additives and salt.

Worry the Proper Way

Worrying is part of human existence, where it becomes an issue is when the person with anxiety disorder worry over issues that are not relevant. The whole essence of treating someone with anxiety disorder is not to completely eliminate the issue of worry since anxiety has its own positive role. By attending to issues quickly and going over the issues can help a person stop themselves from worrying unnecessarily. Have a plan for the week, which is then broken down into daily plans that will help you be in control of things around you.

Join Support Groups and Learn from Others
People with anxiety disorder find out that they are able to understand their condition better if they have access to forums or groups where they meet other people to give and receive support. The interaction with others who also experience anxiety or have gone through a similar path can help reduce the feeling of loneliness and provide the opportunity to learn more about the disorder as well as provide an important social network.

Getting Help, Where to Go
- Support Groups
- A Psychologist
- A Therapist
- A Doctor
- A Counselor
- Health Centre in your Local Community

Alternative Treatments for Anxiety

1. Aromatherapy

Aromatherapy, also known as essential oil therapy is a holistic type of healing that uses extracts from natural plants to treat, promote and improve the physical and mental health of an individual.

Aromatherapy is able to ease stress and anxiety by using its aromatic essential oil to medicinally reduce the heart rate as a short term measure and make the patient find it easier to sleep.

2. Cannabidiol Oil (CBD oil)

CBD oil is a derivative of cannabis or marijuana plants. CBD differs from other forms of marijuana because it does not contain the component of the plants called tetrahydrocannabinol, or THC that causes the senses of the individual to feel high. CBD oil is able to calm down an individual and slow down the process of the person becoming anxious. Although some individuals prefer to take CBD oil as a way of soothing the effects of their daily worries, some others prefer to use it to treat other more serious ailments like generalized anxiety disorder.

CBD Oil is still viewed as a controversial subject and is presently legal only in a handful of states and countries. Laws governing cannabis and other controversial products tend to vary widely from state to state, therefore, it is very important to find out the legality of using CBD Oil in your state before attempting to use it.

3. Herbal Teas

Some herbal teas are able to help remove the effects of occasional stress and anxiety, Most of them work by helping the patient sleep easily. Some teas work by just soothing the person while others are able to have a more direct influence on the brain and alter certain stress hormones. Some type of herbal teas that have been found to be useful include; Chamomile, Peppermint, and Valerian.

4. Herbal Supplements

This is similar to the herbal tea and is believed to be also effective in calming down anxiety.

5. Spending Time with Pets

Many pet lovers know that living with pets has a lot of benefits. Pets provide support, love, and companionship and make the owners healthier. Most people tend to feel happy in the presence of animals and observe that they enjoy a better state of mental and physical health. Common animals used as pets include cats and dogs. By spending some time with animals, a person can also alleviate stress and anxiety.

Natural Products for Anxiety Treatment

If you are someone living with depression, anxiety disorder or post-traumatic stress disorder, then know that you are not alone. About 18.1 percent of Americans suffer from various forms of anxiety disorders, ranging from panic disorder to obsessive-compulsive disorder. They are forms of ailment that can lead to depression, even though it tends to fluctuate from minor discomfort to sometimes uncontrollable panic accompanied by physical symptoms.

The rising cost of therapy and medications used in the treatment and management of anxiety along with its unwanted side effects has made more people seek alternative and complementary ways of treating anxiety.

Most psychological disorders often require long-term treatment in trying to solve the problems.

Most natural form of treatment often provide great relief to anxiety and other psychological diseases. They also offer treatments with far fewer side effects compared to prescription medication. That is why many people now prefer to use alternative and effective natural anxiety treatments to lower the risk of anxiety and also they find it safe to use alongside conventional forms of treatments.

Many of the natural alternatives have to take the patient's type of diets into consideration when taking them. The doctors with alternative therapy experience are able to recommend and show how to use any of these therapies.

Although most herbs are generally believed to be safer than prescription drugs, it is always better to check with your physician before using any of the herbal remedies in the treatment of anxiety particularly if the person is pregnant or breastfeeding.

Most natural herbs are usually organic and tend to have little difficulty in being processed in the body's digestive tract, hearts, and lungs. These natural herbs are:

1. **Passionflower (Passiflora Incarnata)**

The Passion Flower herb is a supplement that has historically been used in the treatment of seizures, hysteria, insomnia, and anxiety. It is a perennial type of vine that climbs and is native to the southeastern part of North America. Although, it is now grown in Europe and other parts of the world. It is very effective to reduce the symptoms of anxiety and equally as useful as some conventional medications.

It is also known to aid in the stomach related gastric cramps, heart palpitations, withdrawal symptoms and reduces sleeplessness as well as helping to calm the nervous system.

Passion flower is not considered safe for women and girls who are pregnant because of the presence of certain chemicals that are capable of making the uterus contract, which can lead to a miscarriage. Breastfeeding mothers are also exempted from taking passion flowers.

One drawback of Passion flower is that it causes drowsiness, nausea, vomiting and rapid heartbeat, which is why it is usually not advisable to take it with prescription medications. It can, however, be combined with other sedative herbs like chamomile, valerian, kava, and skullcap.

Experts believe that it is better not to take passionflower consistently for longer than 6 weeks and also to ensure that the correct dosage is taken.

2. Kava

This plant is native to the Polynesian Islands where it has been used as a ceremonial tea for many centuries. It was first discovered over 300 years ago and is a member of the black pepper family. Kava is a non-addictive product that has the same feel as alcohol and is able to reduce anxiety, improve cognitive functions and aid relaxation.

Kava can be used as a natural alternative to small doses of benzodiazepines and tricyclic antidepressants like Norpramin and Ascendin.

Apart from being highly effective in the treatment of anxiety, they are also used in inducing sleep, which aids relaxation, used as an analgesic and in the treatment of depression. Its unique healing property allows it to be used to relieve pains and relax muscles.

In spite of its many advantages, kava increases the effects of sedatives, alcohol, and tranquilizers, so it is always advisable to take kava with some level of caution and ensure you only take the dosage recommended by a doctor.

Although it is similar to Valium in the treatment of anxiety, unlike Valium it does not reduce cognitive functions.

3. Valerian Root

This herb is a medical root native to Europe and found in some parts of Asia and North America. It is commonly known as a treatment for the sleep-related disorders and has been used for many generations in managing anxiety, mood and other forms of psychological stress.

Its extracts are sometimes found in some food and beverages as flavors. The valerian root is able to increase the number of chemicals called gamma-aminobutyric acid (GABA) that helps in the regulation of nerve cells to reduce anxiety. It also uses some other components that serve as anti-anxiety agents and does not have the kinds of side effects prescription medication that does similar jobs have.

Valerian was widely used during World War I as a tranquilizer in the treatment of soldiers who were affected by shell shock.

Europeans have been using the drug for more than a century to treat menopausal nervous anxiety, hysteria, and irritations.

It is always better to consult your doctor before taking this drug as the dosage and timing for using it as a treatment for insomnia differ when using it for treating anxiety.

The popular Valium drug is derived from this herb and in its traditional form which has a really offensive smell despite its sedative qualities. It is usually not advisable to take the drug for more than 3 weeks because of reported cases of adverse reactions to the use of the drugs which can include apathy, mild depression, and stomachache. Women who are either nursing or are pregnant are also advised not to use this drug in the treatment of anxiety.

4. Lemon Balm

Lemon Balm is an herb that works by calming the body's digestive system as well as reducing the blood pressure of the person. It is also commonly used as a sedative and for many problems associated with the nervous system, stress, depression, headache, palpitation, insomnia, and hysteria

Lemon Balm has been in use for many generations, as far back as the Middle Ages in the reduction of stress, sleep disorder, and anxiety. It has a sweet taste and slightly warming feel which is why it is sold as a tea, capsule, and tincture. The presence of rosmarinic acid gives it the anxiolytic qualities that make it an effective inhibitor of GABA transaminase.

It is often used to improve mood and mental alertness and is sometimes used in combination with other herbs with calming properties like hops, passionflower, valerian and one we will talk about later, chamomile.

Lemon balm can be used by nursing mothers and pregnant women only under the strict supervision of their health practitioner and only when extremely important, otherwise, it should generally be avoided when in such condition.

Lemon Balm is considered generally safe to use, but there have been some reported cases of abdominal pain, vomiting, nausea, and dizziness.

5. L-theanine or Green Tea

Green tea and its supplements tend to come as beverages and filled with many antioxidants useful in the stimulation of the production of GABA used in controlling a major part of the central nervous system. The amino acid in the green tea called L-theanine is what acts as the anti-anxiety remedy, that helps to reduce fatigue, calm minds help the individual relax and can almost be used on its own to treat anxiety.

This L-theanine is also able to curb an individual's heart rate and blood pressure from rising. Green tea is considered generally safe, although some people have been known to experience some form of stomach ache and constipation.

6. B-Complex Vitamins

Balanced diets help to supply the body's needs for vitamins and other nutrients, however, it may sometimes be necessary to take some vitamin supplements like Vitamin B Complex to augment whatever may have been gotten from food. Vitamin B-Complex is commonly found in foods like cereals, grains, seafood, potatoes, eggs, and dairy products. Vitamin B-Complex is very useful in ensuring the energy levels of the body is sustained and contains antidepressants like dopamine and norepinephrine to help reduce the effects of stress, depression, and anxiety.

The B vitamins in the body get burnt up and quickly consumed when the individual is greatly stressed and the process helps to reduce irritation, improves concentration and ensure the nervous system stays healthy.

Vitamin B-Complex, when taken by girls, is known to be easily absorbed by the body and has a very low chance of an overdose with very rare side effects like itching, allergies, and diarrhea. Other symptoms may include some form of heartburn, sunlight sensitivity, skin patches, and nausea.

Vitamin B-Complex is a natural anxiety and stress reducers with calming properties. Many health practitioners consider Vitamin B-Complex as one of the best low-cost natural supplements that are very effective in the management and reduction of anxiety, depression, and stress when compared to the other types of natural supplements used in controlling anxiety.

7. 100% Pure Lavender Oil

This is another effective natural healing remedy that is able to significantly reduce the effect of anxiety and depression in a person, although it is often underrated. The benefits of this oil in overcoming anxiety and depression are gained by rubbing the oil in your palms and using the hands to administer it on the body as a form of massage. That is not all, there are pure Lavender oil candles that can be burnt daily while playing spiritual songs that can be used in relaxing. Some hospitals have caught up with it and are already using it as a natural anti-depressant of choice.

This oil is able to help the body cope better with the daily stress and anxiety and acts as a general tonic in the clarification of the mind, restoring vitality and calming of nerves.

8. Chamomile

This herb is very popular in the suppression of the production and the release of the stress hormones in the body that triggers the anxiety disorder in some people. It is a mild and gentle remedy helps in treating insomnia, gastrointestinal upsets, and anxiety. It has been used for more a thousand years and can even be given to children. Some of the compounds found inside chamomile bind itself to brain receptors in a similar manner to Valium and can be combined with other prescription anti-anxiety medications to increase their efficacy.

In addition to its ability to relieve insomnia and tension, it is also known to improve stomach functions and reduce stomach upset that accompany anxiety.

Chamomile can be consumed in the form of liquid extract, capsule, tablet, tea or supplements. It is not advisable to take this product if the woman is pregnant or breastfeeding and can sometimes have side effects like skin rashes, swellings in the throat, and shortness of breath. It is also observed that people who are sensitive to ragweed, estrogen, marigold, and daisies tend to also be sensitive to this herb.

9. Magnesium and Calcium

Magnesium and Calcium are very important minerals useful in the body. They have also been found to be very good natural remedies for anxiety. The way these two minerals combine to reduce anxiety in the body is quite complimentary, while magnesium acts as a relaxant, calcium tenses, so when the body is tensed, calcium ions are produced that move into the cells of the muscles. Whereas when the person is relaxed, the magnesium helps to remove the calcium ions from the muscle cells to regulate the heart, nerve conduction and contracting of the muscles.

Ironically, the symptoms associated with magnesium deficiency are very similar to those associated with anxiety. They include; fatigue, rapid heartbeat, irritations, numbness, and insomnia, which are the major symptoms of people who suffer from anxiety. However, we must not forget that magnesium always works in combination with calcium to achieve the desired result.

People who suffer from depression or anxiety disorder tend to have excess calcium levels, which mean that the probability of the magnesium level being low is high considering that magnesium and calcium work in tandem.

Magnesium is mostly found in green vegetable, nuts, seeds, beans, spinach, and peas.

10.Omega-3 Fat

Another natural form of anxiety treatment is the use of omega-3 fatty acids, which is perhaps not yet as popular as others. This is because studies are still ongoing and results are only beginning to trickle in, that seems to support the use of omega-3 fatty acids as a form of natural treatment for anxiety and even depression.

In some studies conducted, it was found that those who were given omega-3 fatty acid supplements had a significant reduction in their anxiety symptoms compared to their counterpart who were not fed the supplements.

There are justifiable reasons why it is believed that Omega-3 fatty acids can be used to stem the cause of anxiety. They are known to be anti-inflammatory and able to fight excessive oxidation and are able to boost the production of dopamine and serotonin that ensures that the anxiety levels are kept normal at all times.

Omega-3 fatty acids are mostly in walnuts, sprouts, Brussels, chia and majorly in supplements, tablets, and hemp seeds.

Other Effective Non-Herbal Techniques

Apart from the aforementioned natural forms of remedies, various forms of relaxation, exercising, meditation, and natural sunlight are other proven strategies that are helpful in the reduction of anxiety, depression, and stress.

Meditation can be combined with activities like walking with a great soothing effect on the body. It has the effect of clearing the mind and providing inner peace.

The outdoor experience also provides the opportunity for the individual to interact with others during their visits to the park, garden, and beaches which are also great places where meditation can be practiced. The ambient, scent of flowers, grasses, sounds of birds and even the insects can all contribute to make your day a pleasant one.

Here is One More Thing

If you enjoyed reading this book as much as I have enjoyed writing it, I'd appreciate if you can post a kind review in the comments section.

Your comment can go a long way in convincing someone who is yet to decide.

Your support means a lot to me.

If you want to suggest ways of improvement, you can contact me here.

Thanks once again for taking your time to read this book.

Portia